Coast

Coast

in

6 Days

First published in Great Britain 2013
ISBN: 978-0-9568453-9-9

Published by:
The Wacky Wordshop.
40 Emmerson Way
Hadleigh
Suffolk
IP7 6DJ
http://thewackywordshop.co.uk

For Mum and Dad. All I have ever wanted is for you to be proud of me.

Prologue

"It is not the critic who counts; not the man who points out how the strong man stumbles, or where the doer of deeds could have done them better. The credit belongs to the man who is actually in the arena, whose face is marred by dust and sweat and blood; who strives valiantly; who errs, who comes short again and again, because there is no effort without error and shortcoming; but who does actually strive to do the deeds; who knows great enthusiasms, the great devotions; who spends himself in a worthy cause; who at the best knows in the end the triumph of high achievement, and who at the worst, if he fails, at least fails while daring greatly, so that his place shall never be with those cold and timid souls who neither know victory nor defeat."

Theodore Roosevelt
Citizenship in a Republic
Paris, France on 23 April, 1910

The beginning.

"Five marathons, five days, in five countries. What do you think, Jim?" Spoken with a strong Northern Irish accent by Mark Pollock, my Superintendent at the time. Essentially, I have him to thank … or blame … for what we did next. Mark, like myself, was a Marathon Des Sables veteran. He'd given me help and advice before my race in 2010. I knew he'd a few ideas up his sleeve for a team event in 2011, but the 5x5x5 came as a shock; a welcome one.

I immediately offered my assistance, and began recruiting a potential team to start training as soon as possible. The plan was simple. In one year's time, September 2011, the team would run a marathon somewhere in each of the British Isles and Ireland, finishing in England with the Robin Hood marathon in Nottingham. Following my usual MO (modus operandi) I took on every role from chief organiser, administrator to personal trainer. I didn't mind this, but to do it constantly could cause unnecessary work for me. On this occasion it was one of my better decisions.

Plans progressed rapidly. The final team selection consisted of myself, Mark, George Westoby, Aidy, Bailey, Ben and Ian Wright. The plan was to run a marathon in Scotland, then over to Northern Ireland, on down to Ireland, back across to Wales then finish in Nottingham, England. It all sounded so simple. At a team meeting in our 'local', tasks were agreed and a training programme decided. We'd develop our distance training over the period January through June to achieve, and become comfortable with, running marathon distances (well, as comfortable as could be). This would be verified by running a few races around the May and June period. Thereafter we'd reduce our mileage and start the back-to-back training essential for the daily grind of ultra running.

We decided, as a team, we'd race for a couple of charities. We chose Help for Heroes (H4H) and a local one, The Amazon Breast Support Group based at King's Mill Hospital. We chose H4H because Aidy and I are ex-squaddies. The local cancer charity was chosen to support Angela Norman, one of my police colleagues, off with severe breast cancer at the time; it made things far more pertinent to us.

Training begins

Well, it all began so smoothly. There were no issues. The guys were getting in their regular long runs with no problems and the basic plans of how we were going to execute the event were drawn up. The minibus plus six (runners and support crew), ferries and B&B etc ... no problem, simple ... right? No. Early into the training program Aidy's partner, George, dropped a bombshell ... she was pregnant. I couldn't have been happier for them but I was gutted she wouldn't be coming with us. The strange part is that George was on my team at work, and when she heard about the event she instantly volunteered ... and also volunteered Aidy. Next went Mark. After only a few Sunday runs he discovered his hip was pretty much knackered, so that was him out - a big loss for us.

Belvoir Challenge (March)

So, we were now reduced to a four man team; myself, Aidy, Ian and Ben. We were bonding well as a team and Aidy and I ran the Belvoir Challenge in March, in Leicestershire. It was a hard, wet and muddy 26 mile cross-country route with stiles every bloody 500 yards. But we ran well, looking strong as a team all the way and still finishing in a respectable 4hr 38mins. Looking back, it was a fun race. This was Aidy's first marathon and, I suspect, Ben's, although he maintained otherwise. They'd both run well, keeping a solid pace throughout, brilliant, considering the mud was 3 inches deep all the way. With 50 yards to go I was in hysterics. Aidy, who'd shown no sign of weakness throughout the event, went down with a hamstring cramp. Ben, who'd struggled all day, then popped up bold as brass and said to Aidy - who is trying to run whilst bent double and running parallel to the ground - "You OK, Aidy?" It may not sound funny to the reader, but to Aidy and I it was hilarious. I could see the disbelief in Aidy's eyes - gobsmacked. It was so confident and cocky ... I howled with laughter.

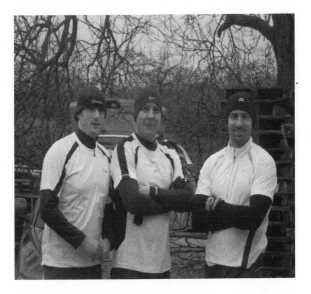

Ben, Aidy and the author on the right,
ready to tackle the Belvoir challenge.

Decision time

Shortly before our next training race - the White Peak marathon - I had to make a big decision, as did the team. Mark, as a police Superintendent, was in a far stronger position to help us obtain donations and sponsorship for our cause. Once he'd left I soon felt the apathy of companies for our cause. The cost of petrol alone would be well over £500.00 and the ferry cost for a minibus plus six amounted to more than £550.00. Once the costs of B&Bs for the team, plus food, snacks and drinks for the week had been calculated, they really piled up. Eventually I did my sums: total costs amounted to just under £3000.00. This wasn't good ... so it was decision time; we couldn't do it, so what now? It didn't take me long to decide.

A year before I'd read an article on some lads who'd run the English 'coast to coast' (west to east), approximately 192 miles in seven days. This worked out around a marathon a day over the seven days rather than the 'five in five' days we'd planned, so the distance and race time were more, but now was an opportunity to change it! I thought to myself, 'How can we push this and how can I push my own limits.' I had done back-to-back marathons in the past, and, selfishly, I took this opportunity to tackle something bigger and better, something special, something that would push my own limits to the max ... so, 'How about doing the 'coast to coast' in six days'? This would be an ultra marathon a day, approx 32-36 miles a day for each of the six days across rough terrain, having to navigate all the way.

I called a team talk to discuss the problem, knowing I had a solution. It was exciting, telling them over coffee at our local Costa. I revealed my idea ... they loved it. I expanded on exactly what we were taking on, and just how much harder it would be than the 5x5x5; the 6x6 would be horrendous. Six ultra marathons in six days would be a massive ask and take a lot more training than originally planned; not only that, but to keep costs down we'd have to rough it. I didn't realise then what problems this would cause. That was it; all agreed; time to plan the route, organise and set up the bigger training schedule. The training plans appear in Appendix A. The overall plan was pretty simple.

January to June we'd build up from 'reasonably comfortable' to marathon distance (it's never comfortable). After a time I would drop the long, weekly distance of 18-20 miles and the speed sessions, and replace them with a reduced distance run of between 8-10 miles, but then introduce back-to-back training. Gradually each week would be built up till eventually we would, by September, be at 20, 20, 23 and 26 miles. This was very gradual but to look at it in my head scared me to death, so I never placed it that far ahead on paper, otherwise I think I'd have lost the entire team! This was a massive undertaking for us, demanding a huge effort from everyone, including families. Due to the high mileage required on the 6x6 I needed to test us to make sure we were capable of doing that kind of daily mileage; not only that, this would - more importantly - confirm that we were capable; mind over matter would play a massive role in this race. To help us with this, I entered us in the Grimsthorpe 70 for the end of August, a 70 mile non-stop race; perfect ... not only physically, but mentally it would confirm that if we could run 70 miles in one day without sleep, we could run it in two days with. But first came the White Peak marathon at the end of May.

White Peak marathon (May)

Five months of training took us up to the White Peak marathon. held in the Derbyshire peak district. Ian couldn't make this again due to shifts, which I think made Aidy and Ben a little nervous as it might be thought he wasn't putting in the miles. I had no worry on that score; I knew he'd be doing the mileage, just alone; either way I knew he'd be fine. Ian had progressed with his training greatly over the past three years. As his best friend and trainer I would have liked to have taken credit for that, but I couldn't because, as it is with most training, it comes from having a strong mindset and the will to push oneself to the max ... every day. This desire to push 'yourself' would prove the most important factor within the team in the months ahead. It would also lead me to discover a lot about myself, my team, and what makes teamwork ... what really drives someone.

Back to the White Peak race. After arriving in the depths of Derbyshire at 6.30am (as I had misread the starting instructions ... that was opening time ... not coach collection time) we registered, then popped to a local cafe for a brew and discussed the day ahead. Aidy, Ben and I were looking forward to the event but Benny kept using comments which were becoming too common for my liking, and which would be used more and more in the coming months, comments that make a trainer or team leader nervous such as: 'We'll just see how it goes', 'We'll just take it steady and walk when we need to'. Erm, no ... this is a race my friend. Ben was nervous - perfectly normal - but I couldn't help feeling annoyed as up to this point he'd been putting in the mileage and doing really well, in some cases better than most of the team. I think overall this was just me being me; I knew he had it in him ... I just wanted him to believe it too.

We started the race on a beautiful sunny day, feeling strong and keeping a good pace which lasted up until about mile 18 or 19. Now, personally, I hated the race up to this point, as I like to be down to single figures and feel like I'm on my way back in. I welcome the pain; it feels like I'm getting fitter ... crazy, I know. Getting to halfway really does my head in as I'm neither here nor there, but at mile 18 I'm counting down to 20, and once in the 20s I feel like the end is nigh ... come on! The pace started to slow, as expected, then came the sudden downfall of Aidy. It was quite amusing really. I had Ben wanting to throw up (due to scoffing energy gel which is of no use to man or beast ... just makes you sick), and whilst trying to explain why he felt sick I heard 'OOOWWW!' I turned round to see Aidy attempting to run bent double again, like at the Belvoir Challenge. It was so funny; he was trying to run with his back parallel to the floor and kicking his legs out at the same time to stop the cramp - like 'The Ministry of Funny Walks' with backache. Ben, who had already slowed right up, then stopped to help Aidy. I screamed: 'NO ... KEEP RUNNING, WE'LL CATCH YOU UP!' I told Aidy to lie on his back whilst I helped him stretch his hams. We caught up to Ben with only a mile to go. There followed 20 minutes of conversation as follows:

Ben: 'I feel sick.'
Me: 'No you don't, you're all right.'
Aidy: 'I can feel cramp coming on again.'
Me: 'No it's not, keep running, you're alright.'

Eventually we saw the end and with only 20 metres to go George and family were in sight. At this stage Aidy got his second wind and went for it with a sprint finish. I remember thinking: 'Where did that come from you cheeky bugger'. In we came, to be greeted with a new race mug and all was done. It had been a hard day in the heat but we'd done it; 3hours 50mins that could easily have been 3hours 30mins; cracking race.

Of the three of us I thought I had come out fine, but a short time later my body reacted to the heat which had been baking my head all day: it decided it to lose half its mass on the toilet for the following half hour. This totally dehydrated me - wore me out. I was shattered, totally out of energy … how I managed to drive home was a mystery to me, and I made it with seconds to spare; I think I actually knocked Hayley, my fiancée, out the way as she greeted me at the door. I learnt something simple; in the sun … wear a hat. After a week in the desert last year, wearing a hat all day, you'd think I'd have known that … wally.

Cheviot Mountain marathon (June)

Marathon training continued up to the end of June, and for me was pencilled in the annual Cheviot 2000 Fell race in Northumberland. This is a 23 mile fell race in and around the Cheviot mountain range which works out to more than 26 miles when measured using a GPS. It's a hard race, going up eleven fells higher than 2000 feet, all beginning at sea level. This race would be a great test for us. Considering what we were setting our sights on, we needed to be smashing this all over.

The race also marked the return of Ian to the racing squad, but we lost Aidy who'd booked a weekend away with the missus (at which he proposed to George ... who said 'Yes'). Ben, Ian and I set off on the Friday afternoon. In between outbursts of torrential rain, typical Northumbria weather, we set up the tent. The forecast for the next 24 hours did not look good.

We went to our usual Italian restaurant in Wooler (The Millan). It was fully booked up till 8.30pm, so we went to registration, thinking we'd eat later. This would prove to be a total cockup on my behalf. After a wait and then registration we spilled into the Italian and ordered lots of red wine, lager, garlic bread, spag bol and deserts. The problem came at about 10.00pm. We'd just finished eating and decided, after a quick pint or two, it was bedtime. Well, I lay there in the tent thinking: '£$%& me, I can't breathe.' Now I know a lot of people are like this, and I'm one; I can't sleep on a full stomach so here lay the problem ... I was stuffed. 11.00pm came, then 12, 1, 2, 3 ... I felt like crying. I just lay there listening to my so-called friends sleep. I say so-called as right then I hated them. I was unbelievably jealous of their sleep. Each time one moved I hoped they'd wake up so I could talk to someone. The closest I got to conversation was around 2.30am when a group of pissed-up people walked past the tent gobbing off. They were that loud I had to stop myself from ripping into them.

Well, 5.00am came and the Wooler Town hall clock struck as my alarm went off. When the boys woke I was already seated upright and right cheesed off. I felt like death and now I had to face running up and down mountains in cold miserable conditions ... this was going to be a bad day. We tucked into our packed breakfasts and cups of tea and made our way to the start line, some twenty minutes away. At 7.20am we were off, team Physwarriors.

The start did not go well. At the start you run down a path for about 150 yards before a sharp right and BAM, up the Cheviot Mountain to 2720ft. It's a God-awful start to any race and soon separates men from boys, as well as your calves from your legs. Your legs and back start screaming at you to stop and you're thinking 'Shit, I've been going for five minutes and I'm blowing, and I've got 5-6 hours left of this if I'm lucky'. I felt dizzy and tired but pushed on, soon leaving Ben behind. He then decided to inform us that he had in fact been suffering with a chest infection for the last few days, but hadn't wanted to let us down. Now, if any of you have ever walked up a mountain - never mind run up one - you will know you need all your strength and lung capacity. Ben had been brave to even start this race, stupid ... yet brave. After about twenty minutes he told me he was going back down. I know he wanted to carry on, but he knew he was holding as back, and that his day would be a bad one if he persisted. I confess trying to keep him going, but we both knew the reality of the situation. It wasn't the race I was concerned about, it was Ben. I recalled how I had felt in the past when I hadn't completed races due to injury etc, and it still bothers me today, in fact it's annoying me now, so I really wanted him to finish. I hoped that he wouldn't be too put off by this and be able to get himself back on the horse ... little did I know what he'd have to push through at a later date.

After we lost Ben we put our 'foot down' and tanked it. All was going well until about three-quarters of the way through when Ian had to catch me before I collapsed after almost passing out from tiredness! Overall we smashed it. The weather turned nasty but didn't stop us. Pushing hard all the way and came in 5th place in 5hours 48mins - awesome! We couldn't have been happier, especially as we narrowly beat another Notts police team to whom I had boasted that we would ... sweet.

The race had not disappointed; as hard as always. Ian and I felt fantastic; we'd pushed the pace all the way stopping only to fill our water bladders then battling the weather; I achieved my best position in the race thus far. We were happy, but next would come the problems and changes in team dynamics I anticipated. I hoped to somehow work around the issues.

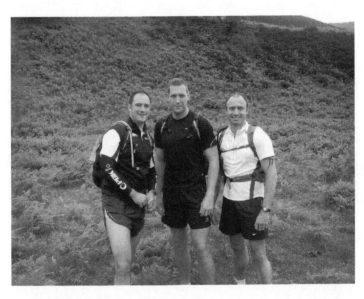

Ben and I now joined by Ian (centre), the start of a long day.

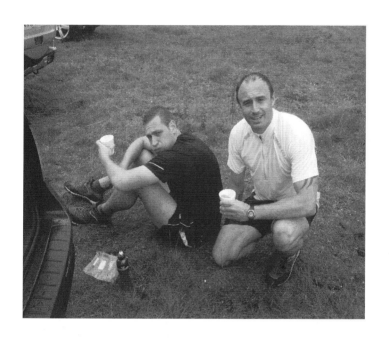

A picture paints a thousand words ... just one
comes to mind for me.

Grimsthorpe 70 (August)

After the Cheviots the team dynamic really did change. Ben started to withdraw from team training, and, more noticeably, started questioning my training strategy - started doing his own thing, i.e. the easy option - cycling. Now I'm not having a go at cycling as, like any endurance sport,its bloody hard, but Ben had a really strong background in cycling, so sloping off for a ride or turbo was his easy option, but wouldn't be mine.

I repeated my call for mileage, mileage, mileage. If you need milk, run to the shop, off to work, run ... it's all time on the legs. Ben ignored my advice. I'd ring him and ask how training was going - usually he'd been out on the bike. I was really hoping he hadn't lost his will to run, which can so easily happen with such a monotonous sport. All runners have been there, whether just starting out or professional ... I just hoped this wasn't his time.

A week after the Cheviots, Ian and I ran the Mansfield half marathon. This was ridiculous. We hadn't rested for more than 6 days and we not only turned up for the Mansfield at 10am, but at 6am we went for a 13 mile run just to increase the mileage; as we would say: 'I'm not getting out of bed for less than 15 miles'. Well, we did the early run around Pleasley and felt okay. After a quick shower and brekky we made our way to Berry Hill and booked in for the 'half'. We both felt alright but Ian really struggled the last few miles. I felt sore but okay. We both finished in a respectable sub-2 hours. Once done I sat down on the grass alongside Ian and his missus, Jacqui. After ten minutes or so I stood up to go home: boom ... knee pain! This was no ordinary knee pain, it really hurt - I was in agony; worrying. A few days later I booked into physio to find out I had massive patella tendonitis and needed rest ... not good.

We continued with team meetings at which I would talk through the following stage of training, for example - the upcoming four to five weeks. By this stage we were achieving some serious distances, as can be seen on the schedule. I had four weeks of not running but worked back up to full mileage mid-July. My knee wasn't right, not the same. It felt weak, just not hurting as much, so it was time to crack on. As I write this section, in January 2012, my right knee is knackered, but the cost of fixing is unrealistic, what with my wedding in 6 months time. Do I rest? Of course I should, do I? No. It's not clever, but it's sometimes harder not to train than train.

Along came August and with it the Grimsthorpe 70, which meant taking into account a week off running - both before the race and after. It would be almost September and the 6x6, so our 70 mile race was essential. In reality it would be our last major training session. As I've said before, I put in the Grimsthorpe 70 as I wanted to test the team physically and mentally for before the 6x6. I believed this to be essential and the lads - apart from Ben - were well up for it. It was his birthday weekend and he wanted to spend it with the wife and little one; I wanted him to run 70 miles. He chose the nice meal with the family. I confess I would have chosen the run (don't tell the missus!) ... but then again I might be an idiot. Now, the 70 was going to be tough. It consisted of 7 x 10 mile laps around the Grimsthorpe Castle estate, starting at 9.00am with a 24 hour limit. I wasn't concerned about the time limit, but I was about the distance - it was a long way. I didn't tell the boys that. I thought that if all else failed I'd let them sleep for an hour or so, but it would all have to go horribly wrong for that to happen. It nearly did.

Unfortunately the race started at 9.00am which meant race registration at 8.00am, with an hour-and-a-half travel time there, plus time for brekky. This meant a 5.30am alarm, usually okay, but then I thought about it. We could be running for 24 hours which meant we could be awake for longer than 28 hours ... mad. Looking back I would probably have camped out on site the night before, but would definitely stop over after the race: why will be explained later.

Well, we lined up for the pre-race photo then at 9.00am we were off. This race would prove to be an amazing experience, but also a bloody miserable one. Obviously we started strong, fighting off the urge to race - easier said than done with Aidy; we could have done with a leash on him.

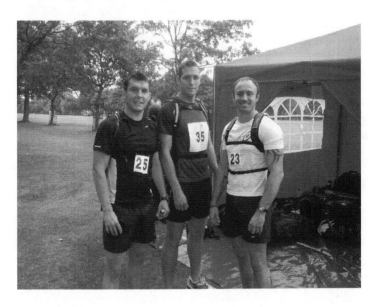

Aidy, Ian and the author

1st lap, yeah, no problem, felt okay but started worrying about the distance. The reason is, you do ten miles and think, 'Yeah... I felt that ... oh dear'. We stopped for 30 seconds, quick snack, then cracked on.

2nd lap, 20 miles down. This time we ate a little more before turning out for lap three as the plan was to get 30 miles under our belts before lunch. Aidy had a quick rub down with the resident physio at 20 miles … his first, and not last, of the day.

3rd lap done, 30 miles down and lunch time: pasta, sausage roll and a brew followed by Aidy having his second rub down with a man he would come quite close to over the next 10 hours. I was pleased to be 30 miles down and actually feeling good. My next mental goal was 50 … and dinner.

4th lap done. Now we were into a brew and snack break at each lap, which was handy for us. We were hungry all the time, and Aidy needed to see his boyfriend in the rub down tent. I would like to say this slowed us down, but in all fairness at 30, 40, 50 miles, we didn't need much excuse for a rest.

5th lap in and the big 50. We debated having dinner at 40, but really wanted only 20 miles - not 30, left after dinner. Amazingly I still felt okay at 50, tired, sore and generally FUBAR … but okay. At this stage I really needed a toilet (tummy) but didn't want to waste time or energy on the 400m round trip walk … 400m, how pathetic. I'd needed to go since about mile 30, and 5-6 hours on I was desperate, but if I didn't want the extra 400m at mile 20 I wouldn't at 50. Fifty was dinner, and what a spread it was. They had a company come in and give us homemade beef stew and fresh bread … man, it was awesome. We all smashed down a bowl or two. Aidy ate fast so he could get back on the couch with his new physio fella, to whom he was becoming very close now, being touched up every 3 hours or so. By this stage they were on first name terms and I may have subjected him to some derogatory comments. Anyway we ate up, had a couple of coffees and after Aidy's rub down were off, two laps remaining … easy … nope!

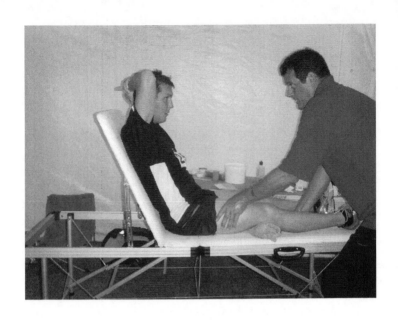

Aidy's new fella.

6th lap. We came in at mile 60 and I felt dead, but after a brew once more ready to crack on to the finish. Aidy's body ruled otherwise; he went down like a sack of sand, fast. He'd seemed normal when we'd first come in, but after a quick sit-down in the tent (it was really cold, dark and wet), he began declining. His eyes started rolling back, his colour went, his speech slurred and his temperature dropped. He started wrapping up, hat, gloves, extra tops - the lot. At one stage Ian and I sat either side of him talking him through the last lap. I know this is cruel, but it was also funny. Aidy was talking to Ian when I asked him something, but instead of turning his head towards me, his whole head fell back and rolled in my direction. As he looked towards me, his eyes rolled and caught up with his head like a slot machine, 'ching, ching ching'. I thought, 'Yep ... he's had enough'. But what I said was, 'You're fine mate, you have a rest and you'll do it'. Aidy was having none of it. He said he was done and told Ian and I to crack on. We sat through 40 minutes to an hour of this before he eventually conceded I was right, and that he would give it a shot; well ... kind of. He started getting his running kit together, at the same time saying to us ... 'I'm done'. Then it all happened. 'Right, I'm ready to go' and boom, projectile vomit everywhere. I couldn't help but laugh and went straight to the kit tent to get his bag so I could get him wrapped up before we cracked on. As soon as he saw the bag he announced he would do it. Over a bloody hour of him saying 'No I can't', and then when he almost collapses it's, 'I'm going on' ... awesome. I think I even tried to put him off, but he wasn't having it. Well, off we went into the night for our 7th and final lap. Now ... at mile 60 I'd felt OK ... shit ... but alright to carry on. Unfortunately, after an hour's rest my body had shut down; it was ready for bed, yet here I was telling it to go again. I felt awful; every ache, pain, knock, bruise, nook and cranny hurt. My stomach felt like a washing machine and my head was already into its sleep cycle ... I was going down.

The pace was slow and Aidy looked like he was at death's door. We went from walk, to tab, to slow jog, and back to walk: a bloody miserable lap, one I'll never forget, even though I try. After about 7 miles in my mouth filled with water and I got that feeling inside which you just know is an early warning that your stomach is about to empty itself. I hastily sat down, waiting for it to pass, but at this stage of the race I didn't think anything could get better, so I cracked on. Eventually, 18 hours 14 minutes later we approached the main drive: what a sight! One hundred metres to go in front of the glorious lit up Grimsthorpe Castle. We crossed the line as a team and after receiving our well deserved medals collapsed into the admin tent.

I felt shocking. After donning some warm kit I had no choice but to start the massive 200 metre journey to the little boys' room. You'd think that after 70 miles it would be easy - oh no! I was dead to say the least. My feet felt like they'd been sanded down and my body like it'd been struck by a car ... repeatedly. The biggest problem was, not only did I know I was going to the toilet, but so did my body. 50 metres to go and I could see the toilet on the other side of a hedge ... bang, it felt like Tyson had punched me in the stomach ... it was coming; 20 metres to go and my trackies were coming down to knee-point in preparation for saving a valuable half second; 2 metres to go - I was reversing at a jog; 250mm to go ... too late!.

Now, if you're a non-runner you may or may not have had this experience, but as a runner, especially a long distance runner, I guarantee that you have. One thing I've learnt from this experience is simple ... if you need to go at 30 ... go at 30! In the belief that the 70 might have taken us less time I'd volunteered to drive us back and drop the lads off at home. Mistake ... a miserable one to say the least!
Within ten minutes of departing, Aidy was in the foetal position, curled up, fast asleep on the back seat, so it came down to my best mate to keep me going.
"Ian ... I'm whacked, stay awake mate and help keep me awake."
"No problem mate." One minute later he was fast asleep, leant so far forward his forehead rested on the gear stick ... great. For the next hour-and-a-half I had to rely on open windows for fresh air and dance about in my seat to some hardcore rave by Scooter, played at full blast. I don't remember much about getting home, apart from a raging pain when my right knee locked up.

Overall, the race had been an amazing achievement, and even if something cropped up to stop us doing the coast to coast I would have still been very happy with this race under my belt for 2011. It gave the team a great mental test, and I felt now that I'd made the right decisions about training, and the race itself. This event could have knackered the lads, or more likely made them see sense, but

knowing how they were they'd realise it would help.
It did. Deep down the lads knew they had, in theory,
run the equivalent of two coast to coast days in one
day, but - during the race week they'd get a nice rest
halfway. I was concerned that Ben hadn't joined us.
This was truly a massive physical and mental test that
had needed doing; it had really helped us. I had
sincerely wanted this to be a full team effort that
would have helped Ben after the
Cheviots. In all fairness - a big ask.

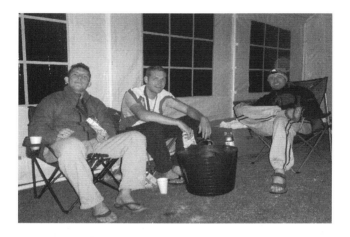

Lovely crisps ... the smiles are all fake.

The Room

Through all our training and races (especially the 70) the boys and I talked about a place called 'The Room'. Looking through my diary entries of the Coast to Coast I don't mention it much, but it took up a major part of our daily chat, 90% of which would be total rubbish.

Now, some people might guess straight away what 'The Room' is, and already have their own personal version of it; some may not. For those who have no idea, 'The Room' is like the 'Wall', only with the 'Wall' you can get over it with some effort, unlike the room, where the effort involved and the overall pain is a whole new kettle of fish. Put it this way, once you have managed to clamber and climb up a hundred 'Walls', you enter ... 'The Room'. Not making sense? I'll try and explain. I suspect that as a team we all pictured it slightly different from one another and I may even one day try and draw it, but for the time being I'll describe it and its relevance to the runner, and me, the writer.

It's a room approximately 6m x 6m square with a normal 8ft high ceiling. It's made sometimes of old stone or old wood depending on how I'm feeling. It does have windows but they're blocked out. In the centre is a small wooden chair - child-sized, not suitable for an adult. In the far corner is a wooden wardrobe consisting of a cupboard at the top and two drawers at the bottom. Inside this room ... is Leroy.

Now, I know what you must be thinking, 'he's crazy', but like I've said before, my diary is what I wrote at the time and the rest of the book is a true reflection of what I thought or of what happened, so as crazy as it seems bear with me, I'm not crazy ... just honest.

Anyway ... where were we? Ah, Leroy. Leroy is roughly 6'5" tall and built like a brick outhouse. He's packed full of muscle, ripped, and can run a sub-3 marathon when it takes his fancy. He's black, wears a tight vest and 'combats' and is a right good looking fella. He's everybody most people are not; your

No. 1 running enemy, your negativity, your weakness, your tiredness, your lack of will, your fear of failure all wrapped up in one good looking package. I know what you're thinking; 'He's crazier than I thought', but bear with me.

On some stages of the Coast to Coast or 70 I'd feel shattered. That's when I'd announce I was 'in the room'. This is where your soul goes when you're FUBAR. If I was to feel merely tired or worn out I might not be in the room, merely looking into the room through the open door. As my tiredness progressed I'd make my way slowly inside before the door was shut and locked behind me. At this stage I'd tell the team - usually after a bout of silence - 'I'm in the room'. They'd instantly know - 'Jim's struggling'. As my fatigue increased I'd move closer to the chair, eventually taking seat. At some stage Leroy would make his appearance. He'd be pleasant at first, right before setting about on a brutal and punishing beating. I may then announce, 'Leroy is kicking the "£$%^ out of me'.

Sometimes, if I'm lucky, I may not be totally dead to the world, just tired enough to want solitude, at which stage I'd go directly to the cupboard. The cupboard is a sad, lonely place. You're in the room, but not taking a beating, just taking five minutes. I sometimes loved it in the cupboard but had to battle my way out more often than not - and quickly! It's not great for team morale when the captain and navigator becomes recluse - then you're in the shoe box, and it's much harder to get out! I'll end this chapter by stating that on the last lap of the 70 miler Aidy was taking more than just a beating from Leroy ... if you get my drift.

Overall training

Other than 'miserable' there is no word to describe the training. That doesn't mean I didn't enjoy it, I did. I can look back with fond memories - one of the joys of pain - you soon forget how bad it was. For the first six months, when training was building us up to marathon standard, the team thought it was rough. It would be nothing compared to what we had to face. We enjoyed it. We got to run in locations we hadn't run in before; Sherwood Forest with Ian, Bolsover with Aidy, Southwell with Ben or Pleasley with me, and it was great. We were getting fitter and bonding as a team in beautiful new areas ... times were good. Mileage covered in these first six months increased to around 21-23 miles on the weekly long-run days, and we ran medium distances and speed work on remaining days to keep us strong, building a good, strong base layer of fitness, finely tuned with a few marathons chucked in.

Once this was completed the real training started. We dropped all the distance off and started a hard regime of 4 days of back-to-back training with three off, starting with short distances and increasing weekly. This was when it got really miserable. Run time increased to two, three, four hours a day. On top of that, add the running prep, and more importantly - the post run collapse. This really increased the daily training session; not easy having worked a 9 hour shift. The worst part of the post run time was the three simple words spoken before you left whosoever's house you'd began running from - 'What time tomorrow?'

Looking back it's amazing the crap we came out with, and what crap still come out with today that we consider normal. Example - the brew situation. After each long run we'd have a cup of tea and a few (in Aidy's case, ten) biscuits. We really enjoyed our brews. It marked the end of our daily grind, but this was the problem ... we REALLY looked forward to our brews, and had somehow developed a rule which forbade any mention of a brew or biscuits before there were less than 30 minutes remaining. God forbid you breached this unwritten code, it was heavily frowned upon. One day on a casual run with the boys we took George (now back fighting fit) for a steady run, and she mentioned she was looking forward to a nice cuppa. This was outrageous behaviour - she was speedily put right.

It's amazing what you put up with and get used to through training. The mind and body are an unbelievable combination that always astounds me. The training was miserable - just one word to describe the most awful pain you can really, lawfully, put yourself through. Once you start hitting big mileage, especially back-to-back work, you raise the pain to a whole new level. Every part of your body aches, your ligaments hurt, your heels are bruised, your skin is raw and you spend hours figuring out ways to avoid that pain next time. You feel this way (when you first start distance running) after a short one hour run, and think to yourself ... 'How on earth am I going to run 10 miles, never mind 26, or 30 odd on the Coast to Coast'. But you can, and you do. That's why we're so unique and amazing; our bodies and minds develop, change according to our situation, and adapt so we can tackle what we next throw at it. We never believe we can actually do more, but when we do we don't seem surprised, we just get on with it. We're truly tremendous machines - sometimes we need to remember that. We soon forget we have done or can do it, especially when, a few months later you return to distance running and struggle with a 1hr 45min run ... you guessed it ... me.

Race organisation

I wrote this chapter at the last minute, having given serious thought to what I would want from this book were I to buy it. I've read similar books in the past because I wanted not only to see how far someone could push themselves, but also to learn how they did it. Many books describe how the writer felt, or where they went, but I wanted detail - ideas and help - on how I could do something like or even better it. Here is an overview of what we did to make it to the start line.

I won't bore you with the original plans for the 5x5x5 as at the time logistics and costs made it unrealistic to pursue, but even so, the 6x6 proved a nightmare to arrange, so I guess rule one of 'how to', is ... be realistic. Beginning early 2011, I convinced the team to give me £10 a week each to accumulate some £600 toward accommodation and food etc. This would prove to be essential and was discussed at one of our early monthly meetings. At the first meeting I allocated roles to the team. This is not the full list, just some of the main jobs needing sorting: food and drink, accommodation, petrol, transportation, sponsorship, training schedules, route finding, first aid kit, media, donations, kit, medals, drivers, support crew, insurance, time off, right through to where we would go out on 'finish night'. This list would grow, mutate and change continually depending on situations, what item worked better, who knew who etc. I immediately knew that organising would be tougher than the training.

The plan

I devised a plan of attack for the six days and planned around it. Using a Harvey's Coast to Coast map I divided the route into roughly six equal days, trying to end each route in an urban area if possible (for amenities), or at least a camp site. Several attempts later it worked out at day 1 - 31.5 miles, day 2 - 32 miles, day 3 - 33.5 miles, day 4 - 34 miles, day 5 - 32 miles and day 6 - 29 miles, total - 192 miles. Once this was done I went about picking the best camp sites or barns I could get, at the cheapest price in those areas, and booking them early for 6 of us.

We were very lucky. I managed to secure a 6 man tent free, from Argos, and Ben secured enough Army ration food to last us all week. I knew that at times the rations would be a bit grim, but it would save us a fortune. Supermarkets also chipped in and after a few trolley dashes we had enough energy drinks, pop, brew, kit and sweets to sustain us for the week. We begged and borrowed all sorts of camping kit to reduce costs, and also managed to borrow a mate's Mercedes C-class 7 seater, although I don't think he's my friend now!

All the above looks easy, but with a full time job, hours of training and a fiancé to keep happy, all of a sudden your spare time is significantly reduced. When you've finished work and your four hour run it's not easy telling your missus you're going online for a couple of hours, sending begging emails or route finding. Eventually I sorted our transport, all our food and drink, a support crew of two and a route. Now it was time for the small things, the fine detail, to make the week go smoothly for the runners, support crew and family at home.

I plotted the route and prepared a laminated route card, along with a map for the support crew. The guide showed every checkpoint we'd visit including grid references, place names and distance in miles between each one. This route card would also be in the spectator guide I produced, for family and friends to follow our daily progress. It would also give them instructions as to where and when to meet for the final leg, and the subsequent (hopefully) celebratory meal (see Appendix B).

First crossed words

I've never been renowned for my soft side, or my ability to keep my mouth shut, which in most instances is good as it gets the job done, but one rule to this is ... know your audience.

Ben did great, securing some donations for us which helped no end with camping and fuel costs. This also caused the first of our many heated discussions. Ben knew the managing directors of two companies he'd approached. One company offered us £1000 and the other offered us £500 towards the costs of the event. This was great; with £1000 I could refund the boys and maybe have some left over to lift the charity money. Ben didn't see it this way. At a full team meeting, including support crew (Sean Brown and Lee Huffer), he immediately said we should book B&Bs rather than camp. I had been forewarned so had done my maths prior to the meeting. Average B&B costs at £35-£40 per night each (£280 per night for seven nights) = £1960, plus fuel - £500, plus £200 for extra food and emergency money etc - totalled some £2660. We had a total of £2100. So the discussion tap-danced around B&Bs and bunk barns. I agreed, yes, we could do it - but I had three issues. This was supposed to be a real test, not just endurance, but living in, and on basics ... roughing it ... it wasn't a holiday. Why spend it just because we have it; we were doing it for charity for crying out loud! We didn't have cash yet anyway, and I wouldn't book anything till I could see the green.

The conversation morphed into argument ... voices soon rose. Ben accused me of not listening to anyone else's opinions. I said I would if it wasn't a stupid idea, and stated: 'This isn't my first rodeo'. Maybe I shouldn't have jumped straight in and rejected the idea outright, but the reason I did what I did, was that I knew it wasn't just Ben speaking, (Browny had been whispering into his ear about it) - he'd mentioned it days before. This was a test of endurance and mental strength. We wanted to rough it, eat ration food and push ourselves to the limit without costing the earth. This was not 'a jolly' and the team and support crew needed to know that. Looking back I now understand I was too harsh with Browny and Ben. I guess I was simply annoyed that not everybody wanted things like I did. In all fairness, I can't blame people for wanting some comfort at night, especially having been 'on the run' for ten hours! Aidy and Ian had no problem with it, we knew that the tougher the week, the better it would feel for finishing it. The meeting ended with the original plan intact, regardless of Browny's crazy ideas about B&Bs in Penrith - about a 40 mile round trip detour. This was for one reason only, so he could have a night out there. This is not the last time the B&B issue would crop up, and when it next did ... BOOM!

The best part is, by the time we got to the race, I think we'd been given a total of £500 from our kind sponsors - a big drop from £1500. Boy, was I glad I hadn't booked us two grand's worth of B&B. I was now learning a lot - fast - about expedition organising. By September we had the camp sites booked, tent packed, transportation sorted, money for fuel banked, food and drink squared away, route planned, the right kit for the job, loads of first aid kit and enough pain killers to knock out an elephant. The only thing left to worry about now was ... were we fit enough?

Here follows a word for word copy of my diary, written each evening whilst slowly dying in the tent, apart from day six ... written a day later.

Sunday 11/09/11
St Bees
Arrival day (St Bees camp site)
22:17hrs

It's 22:17hrs and I'm sat, chilling in the tent. Weather is horrendous but has calmed down a bit now. We put the tent up in the howling wind and rain and I was soaked to the skin. My grey trackies are hung and drying whilst Ben and Aidy sit watching Inglorious Bastards, Lee and Saun are out, supposedly to get us a few drinks in, but that was an hour ago and still no sight nor sound, probably in a curry house.

It took us 5 hours to get here after a very emotional farewell from Hayley. I hate leaving her, I really do. She couldn't even come to the nick for the goodbye but probably for the best, rather say it in private. I miss her already, spent 12% of my battery looking at her pic on my phone 'sat with Loubies (her dog)'. It was a miserable journey up. To say that for the five hours I could just about move my head is no understatement; I was completely covered in kit.

I'm nervous about tomorrow. The severe storm set to hit Britain is one thing, but my bad back and right knee are really on my mind. I could have coped with my knee, but my back is a different matter. It's really worrying me and shows no sign of let up. I feel I can cope with anything, just not my back. But I'll update you tomorrow on that one. Really looking forward to getting tomorrow out the way and getting to the barn, just get day one out the way.

22:38hrs

The boys have returned now with lager and cider in tow, and we're about to toast the week ahead. I really want to be strong this week, I need to be. I'm the leader and have no choice. I like responsibility, I like being the leader, but I'm scared ... but that's good, surely? It's new to me in a different way, leading, planning the whole thing feels good.

I gave a toast tonight ... 'It's going to be miserable, it's going to be hard, but I promise you, the harder this will be, the more amazing you will feel on Saturday'. It's 22:53hrs, time to sign off, boys are just rambling about shit now which is usual, putting the world to rights and all that.

Day 1: Monday 12/09/11
St Bees to Rosthwaite
21:38 hrs
What a day. I'm just sprawled out in my sleeping bag in the Dinah Hoggus Barn in Rosthwaite. Today has been a bloody hard day, harder than I thought. We were up at six, but when I say up, that indicates I was asleep, which is a total lie. Due to the tail end of Hurricane Katia hitting the UK we were greeted and treated to gale force winds all night with heavy rain in the mix, and not just rain - torrential rain all night. I think in total I had approx 30mins. The highlight was going outside for a piss, a bit blustery to say the least. Well, anyway, 6am reveille and got ready for an 8am start. Browny didn't really get the idea of support crew this morning, more like '£$% around'. As a team we need to be more switched on first thing, concentrate on food rather than personal shit. Either way by 8am we were down at the beach of St Bee's with our feet in the sea, posing for pics, and we were off northbound towards St Bee's head before heading east inland for the lakes.

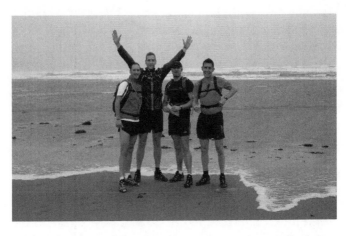

Team pic: the customary dip in the Irish Sea.

Obviously we felt great for the first few miles; Ben coming out with some classic, typically runners quotes like: "Yeah, I'm happy at this pace". (Typical line people say one mile into a 192 mile race!) So usual.

Well, inland we went hitting CP 1 (checkpoint 1) after just 2 hours or so at Cleator (9 miles). Felt ok at this stage and after a quick bite we were on our way. Next CP was only 6 miles at Ennerdale Bridge but £$%$ me it was cheeky over some of the peaks, really took its toll. After some sausage roll and a few crisps we were back on our way for the 12 mile stage to the Slate Mines - an absolute grueller past Ennerdale water and Black Sail Hut YHA. By this stage we were all hungry again and between us had two energy bars to keep us going ... schoolboy error or what?

At the end of the valley we headed NE up Loft Beck between Grey Knotts and Haystacks - a complete bastard. I felt dizzy and sick due to hunger and my back was killing me. I can't begin to describe how ill I felt, and how pissed off I was for such an error. Eventually we stumbled over the top and dropped down to the slate mines visitor centre where, in gale force winds, we ate everything we could get our hands on. I smashed two sausage rolls, several packs of crisps, a pack of tortillas, one coffee and one hot chocolate … amazing.

From here we had a steady 4 mile downhill trundle into Rosthwaite where we found our camping barn. Shit hot! Protein shake, chicken Tikka and pilau rice with lemon sponge pudding … mint. After some admin time, stretching etc, we had a couple of beers in the Riverside bar before I retired at 9.00pm to do my diary. Today was 32 miles in 8 ½ hours. It was "£$$^"£$ miserable and I know tomorrow is going to get worse. All I want to do is crack on, get done and see Hayley on Saturday. I was so excited about ringing her tonight and was gutted by no mobile reception; so, after a return call I spoke to her- it felt great.

I'm shattered and need sleep. I hope I do well tomorrow and keep my mouth shut as I'm already reaching the end of my tether with some people. Today was 33 miles - 8 ½ hours.

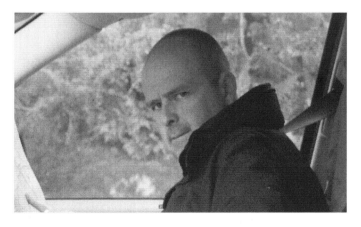

Lee, after only a few hours alone with Browny.

Day 2: Tuesday 13/09/11
Rosthwaite to Shap
22:39hrs
I'm struggling to write this - so, so tired. Up at 6am
as usual and pleased to have had some sleep. Woke
up stiff as a board and quickly got a brew, brekky
(awful fruit muesli) and a selection of paracetamol,
codeine and Ibuprofen down me. We got squared
away and were ready to rock and roll for 8.00am.
Loads more organised today ... so happy about that,
even though Browny came in bladdered. I may have
been half asleep, but I definitely threatened to hit
him.

Today was bloody disgusting, no two ways about
it. We left the barn dead on 8.00am and set off to Mill
Bridge (CP 1, 8 miles) - an awful section. We had to
go up the valley, along Greenup Gill, and over before
dropping back down to the bridge (on the A591). This
section took us bloody hours ... three. It was a
grueller. From there it was straight up and over again
towards Patterdale (CP 2) via Grisedale Tran and
Grisedale Beck. We made great time here and arrived
really early; unfortunately had to wait 45 minutes
for the support crew (SC) - nightmare. Luckily a kind
lady in the village shop let us build a tab up and we
all had a sausage and bacon roll. Oh my God, it was
massive and amazing. Eventually the boys arrived
and after a few minutes for a refill of H20 we were off
on a daunting part of the journey.

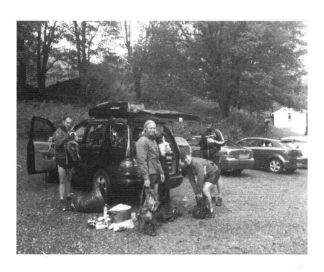

Outside the village shop, ready for the big climb.

The weather now was really shitty, cold and wet, and we had to go up and over again via Angle Tarn before making our way to the Knott (739m) and down to Haweswater via the highest point of the race, Kidsty Pike (780m). This was terrible. Once down to Haweswater (thinking of an easy run into Burnbanks along the lakeside) we began the battle around it. Eventually we pulled into Burnbanks (CP 3) in a bad way, and brewed up. The lads were spot on sorting us out. From here it was only 4 miles to the finish (whatever!). Unfortunately this was across shitty terrain, and being so tired I started cocking up map readings. We got in 11 ½ hours after starting the day and in a completely shit state. Welcome to Shap.

I was gutted and furious to find that our SC had not put up the tent. I almost cried when they announced they'd booked a large room in the farm house for us. Due to doing this for charity, Scott from Newing Farm had given us a massive discount and squared us away with an awesome room for all the team. Showered, carbed and proteined up later we found ourselves downstairs with fresh chicken and bacon pie, new potatoes and veg followed by sticky toffee pudding and a couple of pints of local ale. It was getting on for 11pm - late, but I was soon fast asleep. It had been a most welcome surprise - one I'll never forget.

Today was 33.5 miles, 11 ½ hours.

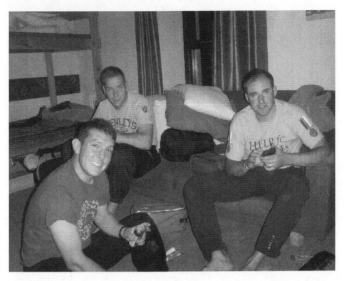

Chilling at Newing Farm house ... a Godsend.

Day 3: Wednesday 14/09/2011
Shap to Keld (34 mile, half way) I woke up, barely able to walk. Pain killers soon became the choice of breakfast along with two bowls of muesli. Photo's etc and at 0805hrs, in good weather, we were off; much the worse for wear, i.e. not walking properly. From here we had a 9 mile leg to Orton which took about 2 hours 20mins. I felt pretty good and Ben stayed up with us ... nearly. He likes to drop back, listen to his headphones and not engage all day. From Orton (CP 1) it was a cheeky 6 miles to Ravenstonedale Moors where the support crew lost us. This caused problems as lack of water and fuel along with another 6 miles to go really hit us. We managed to get hold of the 'grinners' (SC) and arranged to meet at the next CP (they couldn't find CP2).

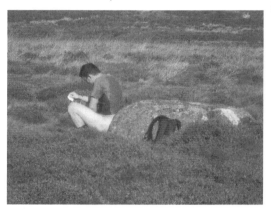

Aidy pauses for a break on the moors.

We arrived in Kirkby Stephen (CP 3) and with Ben having dropped back we started eating rations (mock ham and pasta ... awesome). Ben was clearly struggling but we couldn't go any slower; the day was long enough as it was. Ben then let out about not feeling part of the team. I really struggled not to let rip, considering that he'd ran behind us listening to headphones all day every day. I told him the directions for the next 12 mile road route, and the

43

rest of us went on. This road was shocking, long, hilly, long and hilly (times two for good measure). We arrived in Keld, FUBAR but with the tent already up, and great weather. Another 33 ½ miles down (98 miles for the week). I feel very sore, my knees are falling apart and feet are very painful. I feel fit enough to carry on and of course I will, but bloody hell it's gonna hurt tomorrow. I'm going for the 36 mile option, as I'd planned to stop at Streetlam (34 miles) but I'm going to carry on to the campsite at Danby Wiske. It's a massive ask but we'll do it, I know we will, and I'll write about it tomorrow.

Dinner! Awesome ... chilli and rice pudding ... amazing. I've learned a lot about myself this week, along with team dynamics ... a lot about team dynamics! Pick your team wisely. Any doubts, get rid of; members must be 100% committed at all times, including to meetings, sponsors, and training etc. Pick your support crew equally carefully. You need positivity, creativity and a 'get on with it' attitude; no selfishness. With hindsight, I didn't do either of these properly but I won't repeat the mistake. You also have to be prepared to hurt people's feelings, because when the chips are down and you're exhausted, trying to sort yourself out, there's no time for charity. It's 22:06 and bedtime. So tired, hope I feel ok in the morning.

Today was 9 hours (34 miles).

Day 4: Thursday 15/09/2011
Keld to Danby Wiske (36 miles)
Well, what a day. Awake about 5.00am, waiting for the alarm to go off at 6.00am. Had an 'all day breakfast', tea, coffee and pack of biscuits, then away for 8am. Just the three of us today. Ben was in total agony with his ankles and could barely walk first thing. I didn't know what to say really. I know he was in bad shape but didn't offer to help as I really couldn't do anything. It put a 'downer' on the team. I asked him if he was sure, but deep down I knew it was for the best.

Well, the route start was disgusting, and we spent the next three hours climbing over the moors to get to Reeth (CP 1). It was shite; bloody gorse bush for hours. We finally arrived in Reeth for hot chocolate, coffee, sausage rolls (fresh ones today) and biscuits. I was FUBAR already (after only one leg) as we set off for Richmond (CP2) - another long checkpoint (10.5 miles) and again it really did us. We arrived with Ian in a shit state, having pulled a muscle in his left quad. We had a good lunch at this CP (mock ham again), biscuits, coffee etc, then we were off for Bolton-On-Swale. This was only 7 ½ miles (previous being 11 and 10 ½ mile) but it killed us. It was turning into a hot day and when we got there ... again, no SC. For "£$^ sake! 20 minutes later they arrived blaming 'traffic'. What a load of rubbish!. We later found out that Browny had been looking for a B&B and had got talking (Brownagram ... he's famous for them).

Anyway, this was our last CP so we then set off for our last 7 miler to Danby Wiske. This required a lot of road work - including a long 2-3 mile walk - as Aidy was 'going down' and Ian couldn't walk. Amazingly I felt OK, FUBAR but ok. We arrived at the White Swan PH campsite totally exhausted, mentally drained, to find the tent up ... and nobody home. We'd been out for 10 ½ hours, run 36 miles and were totally cheesed off. Aidy was going down and I was dead. Eventually I got Lee on the phone; he said they were all out -

bloody three of them - looking for a towel to dry the tent ... I thought I was going to pop! Eventually they arrived and before I had chance to say anything, Aidy ripped into Browny, and rightly so. Browny stormed off threatening to go home. It transpires that:

1. They were late for CP3 due to Browny looking for a B&B for himself and Ben
2. They'd gone out again later ... bloody three of them ... so Browny could try again find a B&B. What a nightmare. We had no kit, no food ready, no electric or anything. Thank God Lee gave us a dig out and squared us away, but I still wished Ben had stayed as he had a good idea of what we'd need. Anyway, I felt shit and eventually sorted myself out (shower, food etc). Browny finally, and thankfully, returned ... after trying to ring his missus for a lift home ... think she told him to "£$% off: and I could picture Leanne doing that.
Going to bed early, 36 miles, 10 ½ hours.

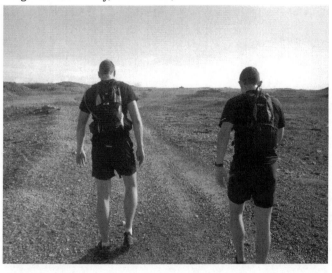

Crossing the lunar landscape on route to Reath, commonly known as Melbecks Moor.

Day 5: Friday 16/09/2011
Danby Wiske to The Lion Inn (30 miles)
I slept OK last night, very quiet ... thank goodness, although it pissed down all night. Woke up at 3.00am and 5.00am for peoples' piss visits; the zip in a tent is the loudest thing in the world. We were up at 6.00am. Browny refused to get out of bed and help (not surprised) but either way we were off at 8.00am as planned, thanks to Lee. My achilles was absolutely FUBAR, tight as hell, so tight it worried me. Ben didn't run again today, still in agony with his ankles, I just hope it's not permanent.

Thank goodness we'd pushed on to Danby Wiske last night; it took 2 miles off our total today. The first 7.5 miles flew by and we got into CP1, near Renny Farm, in 1hr 37mins, amazing; God knows how. CP2 took a little longer but we got in to Swainby in about 1hr 45mins; 14 ½ miles done while feeling shit. We were all struggling by this point. The best thing was, I had set the checkpoint at CP2 as a TK (telephone kiosk) on Hollin Hill; fine for me with my map, but the map I'd given the SC was slightly (and I mean slightly) newer (3 months), and without the TK on it. They spent half-an-hour looking on their map for the TK I had given with the grid reference and had driven all over looking for it before asking a local, who informed them that the TK had been removed over 6 years ago; been replaced with an apple tree. Either way, CP2 was at the side of the apple tree.

From CP2 to 3 was only another 7 miles but £"$^ me it was hard. The muscles were running on empty and we all struggled. Now we really started to dig in, as deep down we knew this was the day to get done as we'd do anything on the last day to finish ... anything.

CP3 seemed like an eternity. Both Ian and Aidy were suffering severely with pulled inner quads, and they couldn't manage the impact of the downhill sections. This really slowed us down as I couldn't even get fast tab on downhill, more like an Adams family Lurch walk, or dragging the injured leg behind like Egor.

We dropped down to the B1257 and found the SC parked on the laybye directly on the C2C route, spot on. We sat chilling for a while; I fought to get a mock ham and pasta ration pack down me along with a few pistachios and the usual hot chocolate and coffee. I struggled to eat and as we were quite high up I got a chill: even with my warm kit on I started going down, and quick. We soon got going after I'd stripped back to shirt and shorts (never start with your jacket on, it will soon be off).

I knew we had a couple of good climbs ahead but once out the way we'd be pretty much level on the moors, but still very exposed. I briefed the team and off we went, before long contouring at about 400m. This section felt like forever, with some really long paths and multiple valleys to skirt, all the while exposed to the elements from on high. Visibility was not great and a hard wind bit into our faces for hours. Just our luck - as soon as we got high, the wind direction turned into our faces.

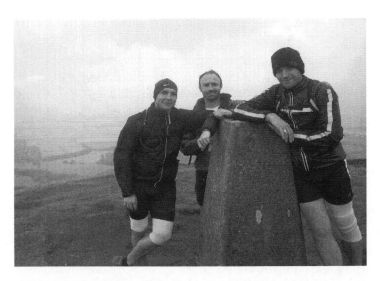

Round Hill at 454m. On route to Lion Inn.

We began really struggling and as the pace slowed, so did our distance covered. Usually after an hour I could show or tell the team we had covered X number of miles, say 5 or 6, but at this stage we were only covering a few Km squares on the map and not getting anywhere. I knew the boys were getting tired. We all felt worn out and I kept trying to keep morale up by explaining how nice the Lion Inn pub was and how we deserved a couple of pints. The pub description got Ian salivating. ""£$^ it, we're having a pub meal tonight ... we've earned it". To which I replied (obviously not taking advantage of a poor little tired soldier slightly delirious through pain and fatigue), "You buying?"

"Yep." Bonus!

Time ticked on and eventually we turned a corner from where I could see the Lion Inn. What a sight for sore eyes. I confess, it did look a distance away, at the end of a large valley, but I would never admit it. I literally felt and saw Ian's last bit of morale desert him at the sight of the distant CP.

"It's "£$^ miles away."

I tried explaining it was only 15 minutes away, but it was no use - even though I was right - which actually shocked me. I knew it looked further than it was, but when you're exhausted, rationale and experience desert you. As we approached it, Ian came out with a belter.

"Looks a bit small."

"That's the shed Ian, the pub's on the other side." Classic Ian. Aidy found this hilarious and after a quick 5 minute climb we were greeted by the front of the pub, and our 6 man tent up and tucked nicely in alongside the pub out of the wind, with electric hooked up. What an amazing sight. After worrying all day, it was up; it couldn't have been better placed. Browny had cheered up, no doubt proud of obtaining the electric hook-up I hadn't booked (I'd been told we couldn't have it, but luckily in getting this spot next to the pub they were able to sort it out). If we were down on the field as planned, it would have been a bloody rough, cold, wet and windy night. In fact, windy wouldn't be the word. It was gale force when we arrived and it just got worse.

Well, into the tent we went and the fallout of the night before must have done the trick; the SC was spot on. The tent couldn't have been pitched better out the wind, electric hook up in; snug as a bug. Hats off to them, Lee, Browny and Ben had done us proud. I felt totally spent but brill, as here we were, one day left, no major injuries and in a tent outside a beautiful pub in the middle of nowhere.

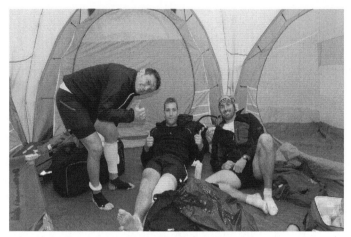

Best tent pitch yet.

After a quick shower in the pub, which included a race to the showers through the main restaurant with shorts, T shirt and towel on, I was clean(-ish) and ready for Ian's dinner. We'd polished off our protein shakes and energy drinks, cleaned up and were ready for an awesome dinner.

I had a chicken goujon starter, which was amazing, followed by a home-made steak and ale pie - bloody lovely - but, due to our slightly shrunken stomachs I couldn't manage it all. Worse, I could only manage one pint of Theakstones black before I had to retire for the evening. Now for those that don't know me, that's a first ... I must have been really tired.

It was hammering it down with rain during dinner but luckily there came a clear patch so, using my remaining battery on the phone I'd broken, I rang Hayley. It felt great to ring and tell her I'd be seeing her next afternoon. We could have talked for ages but I was freezing so with only 15% of battery life left we called it a night: I'd need that 15% for the finish.

From then on it pissed down again but once in my pit I was gone - obviously after my night time complementary paracetamol and codeine tablets. All three of us tried catching up on our diaries but at 9.30pm I was head butting my diary before I gave up. Bed felt sweet and I barely stirred when Browny stumbled in about 10.30pm, pissed up on three pints ... usual.

Today was approximately 30 miles and took us about 8 ½ hours.

Day 6: Saturday 17/09/2011
Lion Inn to Robin Hoods Bay

We all slept well last night, with a little wind and rain, but pretty calm apart from that. I woke up with legs in usual agony. I can cope with sore muscles, joints etc but my bloody achilles were screaming. I struggled to stand; my ankles wouldn't bend and once they started to it felt like they were snapping.

For breakfast it was sausage and beans from a tin, cooked up in the billy can. I felt jealous. I'm sure Ian got more sausages than me, in fact I'm positive. Next stage was the toilet stop. Unfortunately the toilets were inside the pub bar area, which didn't open its doors until 7.00am, the time we wanted to be setting off. It was our last day and we wanted to arrive at Robin Hoods bay at a reasonable time to see friends and family, so we rose at five to be away for seven, hence our dilemma. Wait until 7.00am and rush to get going (if they do open for dead on 7), or take some tissue and find a private spot on the moors. We opted for option 2.

Praising my luck for no rain I went in search of hallowed ground. Now, this is easier said than done, trying to find a quiet spot on the moors out the wind, where people won't tread, yet only a short distance away. As you can barely walk it's a task in itself. Well, off in my sandals I went in the pitch dark and howling winds up a small hill to a wall which had an 'untrodden' look about it. Tucked behind this wall I squatted down in the most uncomfortable position ever. Bloody hell, I was glad that was over; for future reference, remember your head torch. I had sapped all my strength just squatting for two minutes. This was not looking good; the 40m walk had about killed me. Back in the tent we sorted our kit while I planned the route across the moors in my head, to get a bearing on where we were going. Today we'd be joined again by Ben. I didn't think this was the best idea as 1) I couldn't see the point, him having missed two days and 2) he was struggling with the mileage and clearly still in a lot of pain. I can see why he wanted to do it, I just didn't want him making a mess of himself ... although I'd do the same. Well, shortly before 7.00am we had a team photo with the Help for Heroes banner on the motor, then we were off across the cold mist, deep into the North Yorkshire moors. We struggled to get moving but luckily the terrain was flat-ish, so we eventually got a good shuffle going.

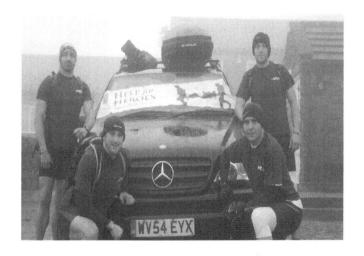

Last day ... come on!

Once across the moors we dropped into Glaisdale for our first CP at about mile 9. En route into CP1 I felt my outer left quad really start to pull, for no reason other than fatigue. It worsened rapidly and I started feeling a little of what Aidy and Ian had felt. By the time I'd come down the hill into Glaisdale train station I was in rag order. After a few minutes I asked for any volunteer who'd like to help me sort my quad out ... bloody hell I've never seen Aidy volunteer so quickly for anything. I think he even put his hand up, like in school ... 'me sir'. Not surprised though, seeing as for the past three days I'd been causing these boys agony - massaging their injured quads. Two minutes later I was lying on the grass verge at

the CP, Aidy pushing his hand into my quad - "£$%
me it hurt. Browny managed to film it all, and I now
know exactly what I'd been putting the boys through.
We didn't hang around too long but we definitely felt
the stop. Ben had struggled to keep up with us across
the moors to CP 1, and I was hoping he'd retire - we
couldn't keep stopping. I knew that once we started
hitting the towns it would be harder with the con-
stant changes in direction, and all the time he was
potentially injuring himself further. But credit where
credit is due, he didn't give up, and off we went
through some beautiful towns such as Egton Bridge
and Grosmont, where we really started to lose him,
waiting for ages in the cold and pouring rain ...
bloody frustrating, because we were running and he
was walking.

On one particular long, road section uphill to CP2
on Sleights Moor, we stopped for a couple of pics,
with the Dad in his RV, of a solo coast to coaster
who'd been with us almost all the way. Eventually
we set off for the CP (not far off) to find the SC with
George (Aidy's missus) and his newborn
daughter Darcie (born the week before we'd left).
George came running up to Aidy in tears so I grabbed
her for a comedy hug, reassuring her I was here. She
was in proper tears; Aidy followed suit when he saw
his baby girl.

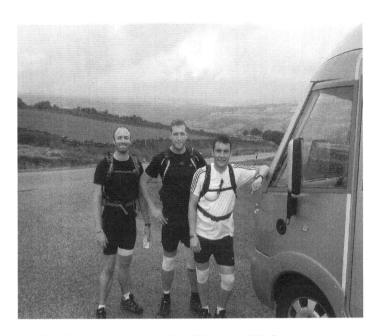

Sleights Moor with the RV, near CP 2.

About 15–20mins later Ben came past and without saying a word grabbed a map and stormed off. I chased after him and had a quick chat; he'd just wanted to get on with it … he knew he was struggling. I made sure he was happy with where he was headed and off he went. From CP2 we crossed a lot of moorland and passed Littlebeck, eventually making our way to Fylingthorpe. Now, this was a slightly different route but we needed one to be sure of meeting up with Ben as the plan was to get there, have a brew and wait for him to catch up, then run in the last 2 miles together. The route looks slightly shorter on the map, cutting through to Fylingthorpe from the A171 instead of going north and down the bay, but bloody hell - I can see why Wainwright chose his route, rather than the two hour slog we took up the hills. As we approached CP3 at Fylingthorpe I was looking down from a steep hill over the small hamlet across to the bay when I got onto my walkie-talkie to speak to Lee, expecting him to be parked up somewhere at the bottom. As clear reception as it had ever been, Lee reported that he was in the bay, and it looked like everybody was there, so we'd better get in. I asked where Ben was; he said he had been picked up. Well, that was it. I looked at Aidy ... think I almost burst into tears. Weather was glorious and we were on top of a hill overlooking the bay - only 20 minutes away. I looked at Aidy and must have said without speaking, "This is it then". It was like a silent conversation between us all. We all knew what we were thinking. Suddenly it hit me; down this hill through Fylingthorpe and we'd drop down into the bay where all this would be over, all the pain from running, all the map reading, all the worry about food, water, CPs, campsites, weather, injuries. Everything would be over, we'd have covered the Coast to Coast in 6 days. That was it! The boys found new energy.

Off we went down the hill, like professional runners, fresh and ready for anything. This stopped abruptly the instant we hit the bottom and faced another demoralising hill. Once up, we hit a main road, the B1447, and for the final time (even though I think he'd not once believed me!) I told Ian how far we had to go.

"Which way mate?"

"Right, mate, then down the hill into the bay, about 700m."

"REALLY?"

"Yeah, just down the hill." Now, this was amazing. Looking at the map I could barely believe it myself. We ran down the road, past the two main car parks on the right, and got to the mini roundabout marking the final 200m downhill section to the finishing stretch. Down we went. A final radio check with Lee stated: "Lots of people here boys, you better be running in." Oh boy, did we intend to. Descending the last steep hill, the bay in sight, we were greeted by a massive crowd and a banner reading:

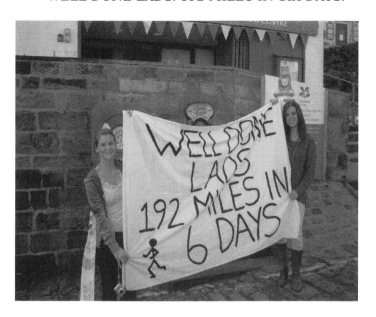

Jacqui and Hayley.

Either side of the banner stood Hayley and Jacqui, and a massive lineup of people clapping us in. I couldn't believe it, it was amazing; there must have been 40 family and friends with another 40 or so locals and holiday makers just out to see these lunatics were who'd run the Coast to Coast in six days.

As we reached the banner, Hayley stepped to one side, so we all stopped running. This drew a loud shout of "Keep going". I'd forgotten that I'd organised some finish tape to be placed near the beach entrance, so off we went again for another few metres. Aidy and Ian ran under it and I snapped it. That was it ... job done.

I looked around to find my Mum putting Help for Heroes medals around the boys' necks, and at last I bowed my head for mine. When Hayley had told me that H4H had sent some medals through the post I

57

hadn't thought they'd be that good: but they were quality, proper job, my mum loved it.

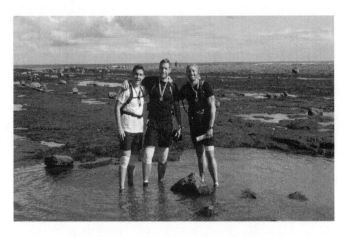

Dipping our feet in the North Sea.

I found Hayley straight away and gave her a big hug. She did well not to cry; I could see she was trying her best. I then did my best to shake hands and hug everyone in sight. Families who I'd no idea would be coming had turned up, and everyone got a sweaty handshake or hug. Five minutes later I heard the shout 'Speech'. Once everyone had gathered around I broke into the speech I'd thought about and planned for months. I'd intended thanking friends and family, support crew, the boys and finally loved ones, who'd put up with us. I'd planned on thanking each one, with a round of applause for each. I'd also prepared a cracking one liner about 'never thinking I'd be happy to see Browny four times a day'. In the end it all went to ratshit; what came out was a thanks to family, support crew and a round of applause. The instant I mentioned loved ones I felt my voice quiver and my eyes fill up. I quickly moved on, thanked the lads, gave them another medal and I was done.

It was great to see all my family and friends together talking. They were all so proud of us; even random people approached me, hugged me, shook my hand, congratulated me and stuck money and cheques in my hand for our charities. I think we ended up with about £65 just from the finish. From here I did the rounds again of handshakes and a little chat with each one, thanking them etc and lapping up the praise. It felt amazing, and I couldn't come down from how good I felt, apart from my knees, hips, back and achilles which all felt like they'd been run over, but, overall - I felt fantastic. I kept close to Hayley and she looked after me, especially by getting us all some chips. Oh, they were good; fresh seaside chips after a day of energy bars, hot chocolate and sausage rolls. After a pint of cider outside The Bay Hotel, loads of pics and some team shots next to the Mercedes SC vehicle and Bay Hotel official finish sign we finally left to clock into our B&Bs and get ready for a meal at the famous Trenchers Fish bar in Whitby. This is where my fine planning and execution of the event went to rat shit!

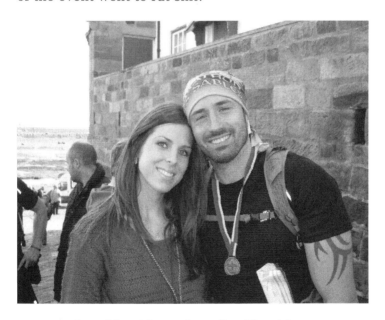

I could not have done it without her.

I stumbled up to the car park with Hayley, eventually finding the Merc keys, hidden under the wheel, and off we went in search of our B&B in Whitby. It took a while; the expensive, all singing and dancing, Mercedes Benz C class was stuck in 1st gear. We arrived slightly early and whilst waiting I started sorting out the car and kit, what a bloody state, it stank.

At 4.00pm the owner, dressed in Gypsy fancy dress, turned up. Hayley went inside to sort out the room whilst I got the bags out. Two minutes later she came back out with a look on her face which said 'I don't know what to do'. The Gypsy stated she'd contacted me ages ago and cancelled our room. Rubbish, all I'd received was a confirmation email. Well, either way there were no spaces available, and realising she'd messed up, sent us to a friend of hers. It got worse; after an hour of waiting and ringing the mobile number on the B&B door the owner rang me back to say she'd not be back till half six. Now, this may be a struggle considering we were due at Trenchers fish bar at 6.45pm! I'd had enough! It dawned on me that my Mum and Dad were booked into a cottage in Robin Hoods Bay, and a month before had offered us a room for free. We'd declined the offer as we wanted the weekend to be a holiday for us and booked the B&B. Another long, slow limp back to the bay at 15mph and £5 car parking charges later I was carrying our bags down the steep hill to the cottage. Obviously I forgot something so had to tramp back up the hill again, after a fashion. I could barely walk and looked an idiot trying to. I finally stepped in the shower at 6.30pm and the taxi picked us up at 6.40pm. At 7.00pm I finally sat down and tucked into fresh fish and chips at Trenchers.

Obviously I'd had intentions (as we all did) of 'getting on it' in celebration of our personal feat of endurance. No chance! Two half-ciders later I was ready for bed. In preparation of making a night of it I'd contacted the taxi firm early doors and asked for a later taxi ... half ten. By 9.00pm I was back on the phone ... 'ten please'.

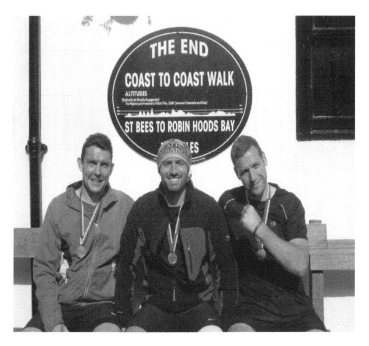

The boys done good, all seated, with the plaque
outside the Bay Hotel.

Looking back.

The day after ...

The following day proved to be a nightmare. My plan
for a day with Hayley, walking the coast of Whitby
after a spot of breakfast and team lunch, turned sour.
To keep it simple, we spent the day in a car park
waiting for a breakdown and then recovery
vehicle before a 4 ½ hour journey back in traffic. A
lazy day's holiday relaxing by the coast had turned
into the hardest day yet. By 9.30pm we were home
and I was happy to be in my own bed, relieved to be
home, and knowing we'd succeeded.

The Ben Situation

I was, and still am, genuinely gutted we didn't have Ben with us all the way. I've thought about him a lot since I got back, mainly because writing this diary has compelled me to debate it with myself. I think Ben will be the first to admit - he didn't put in enough training in and therefore, after three heroic days, putting in a hundred miler, more than he has ever done by a long, long way - he stopped; excessive pain and injury had left him no alternative.

Dealing with pain is just another part of training. It's not all about developing your muscles and CV to cope with the daily grind; it's just as important to train your ligaments, joints (and mind) to put up with it. Without this, by day 2 they will scream at you to stop; they are simply not accustomed to it. But more important than the physicality of it, it was, and probably still is, my personal feeling on the whole situation.

Others may not admit it, or to others, but I know that deep down Aidy and Ian felt the same as me … I hadn't wanted Ben to succeed! This sounds really harsh, and I do feel bad for feeling it, but I stand by it three weeks later as I write. The reason is - I really pushed myself. Every day I'd get up, knackered, and either sit and plan the long route for the day, or wearily get in my car and make my way to Aidy's or Ian's and repeat the process again and again. Every day, mentally prepare for the 3-4 hour run ahead, deciding on how much water, how much dilute, what flavour, which pack, which bottle, what food; take a banana, had a good enough shit or was it rabbit tods (very important!), take gloves, long or short sleeve, trail or road trainers ..? On and on and on and on. And that's just pre-run! Then we get onto the actual, mostly always miserable, long run; knowing that a massive bloody hill in front has to be mastered; that a dug up muddy field has to be run through, that a long, straight, road section has to be conquered, and on and on and on …

If this isn't bad enough - there is the post-run to deal with. Do I have enough time for a brew, a proper stretch, when's dinner, what shall I eat considering today's run and tomorrow's, what time do I start work, can I run on less than four hours sleep, what's that dodgy ankle doing now, what's that niggle in my knee, what on earth is going on with my back and worst of all, the killer, the nail in the coffin ... what time we meeting tomorrow?

So, back to Ben. Why did I (or us) want him to fail? The reason is all of the above. I (we) endured all this daily, put in the miles, banged out the races and then banged out more mileage for good measure. I devoted all my time to either preparing lads for the daily run or race, or planning the coast to coast ... Ben didn't.

I was the one who told the boys that to succeed in this event, 'this is what you'll have to do'. You'll have to do A, B and C everyday. This is your schedule (which you can see at the back). I promised them that if they did as I said, 'You will succeed'; if you don't, 'You will fail'. This was me as the personal trainer, coach, leader, planner and friend telling them how it was - based on personal experience and knowledge. Now, how would I look if Ben, who'd done nowhere near the amount of training we'd done, and no back-to-back training, succeeded? They would think, 'Hang on Jim, I put my life (and family's life) on hold for nine months because you said this is what I needed to do or I'd fail, but Ben has done his own thing; the weekly 13-15 miler and a few sessions on the turbo trainer and achieved the same as us'.

This was the 'vibe' I felt during the event. It was never spoken about, really, but I knew what they were thinking, and I know it's not nice, but like I said, on these events you can't hide from yourself; how you think and feel will come out. I genuinely felt gutted for Ben. His face - when we'd all finished at the Bay - said it all; he was thoroughly gutted. You could see he was wishing he'd followed the training so he could be relishing the experience with us. He believed his failure would affect everything in his life, and perhaps it would. I truly hope he can move on, and I hope we still remain friends. To him, I came across as a bastard, uncaring, unsympathetic and oblivious to his feelings. But I wasn't, I simply had enough on my hands trying to look after myself. At the end of the day, I'm the race organiser, I'm the trainer. It was my event to plan and execute, and if anything went wrong, be it within training, racing or logistics, it was my fault. The fact remains - likely due to a busy family life (which the rest of the team didn't have) - Ben didn't, or couldn't, put in the amount of training required for such an event. I gave him ample opportunity to withdraw, on occasion making it obvious I doubted his fitness. Nevertheless, he turned out and ran three ultra marathons in three days having never run more than 26 miles, and never running more than one day at a time. This was, and still is, a massive achievement for him, and he should rightly be proud of what he did ... because I am.

'So what's next?'

Within two weeks I'd received a call from Aidy - and those were his first words to me. He went on to explain he couldn't actually afford any massive multi-day events abroad, but that I needed to think of something for us to do. As I write this book in October, two months later, I have decided not to think too much about it, deciding rather to enjoy more training for a while, cut back the mileage, run when I want, hit the gym when I want or anything completely different for a change. I'd like to say I'll debate it over Christmas and New Year and start afresh next year, but I've learned over the years I'm useless at rest periods or having no goal. The main reason not to debate it now is, if I do I'll just end up entering myself into an event and going back into daft mileage again. In saying that, it's all rubbish really - thinking about it, I've already booked into the hardest assault course on earth race again - The Toughguy - with the boys ... in January!

The end.

Three weeks later as I write this I question my tone and the words I have used, especially with regard to friends of mine. The thing about challenges like this is that there is no escape, no bullshitting, no hiding, and no falsities. Whoever you are, whatever you're made of will come out on display for all to see, all your strengths, weaknesses, pros, cons, all your good, and definitely all your bad. Your team (and yourself) will see the true you and they might not like what they see, and more importantly, neither might you. Looking back I'm really pleased with my performance. I felt strong when I needed to and suffered when I should have ... daily! At the end of the day, I got the team from point A to point B in the time set, hitting every checkpoint according to plan, and along the way we raised £6000 for charity. Just as importantly, I gave friends who'd never done anything like that before, a massive taste of achievement, changing their lives forever. This might sound a bit much, but ask people who have done anything like this, any major endurance event - they'll tell you they'll never forget it, and once they know they can achieve that ... they know they can achieve anything.

'Carpe Diem'

Acknowledgements.

I cannot leave without a few well deserved acknowledgements. Without help from these people or companies we'd have never made it to the start line.

Firstly, I would thank those companies who helped us with raffle prizes, money and kit for the event:
Mansfield locksmiths who kindly struck medals for the team, putting in great effort in and really making it special - thank you.
Sainsbury's for a trolley full of food and drink - thank you.
To Nick, Browns Bar and restaurant and Brown Beauty for raffle prizes of dinner and makeovers, thank you Dean.
Why Not restaurant for a raffle dinner (love you Johno).
Argos who kindly donated an amazing 6 man tent ... brilliant, thank you Sandra.
To Costa for 52 free coffees (thanks John, I was so desperate for this prize I bought it off the winner).
To Burton menswear for a £30 voucher.
Nottingham Forest for a signed football shirt.
Berghaus, Lowe Alpine, North Face and Crag Hoppers for the raffle kit and clothing, awesome ... I wanted it all.
Thorntons, Mansfield for a big box of chocolates.
Fitness First gym membership for 2 months, Oasis gym membership for 2, Superbowl family pass.
Naaz Indian restaurant voucher (Thanks Royce).
Weekend family pass for Center parcs Sherwood Forest.
Mansfield Electrolysis beauty voucher (thanks Ian's Aunty).
Nibble Me, Mansfield foot clinic voucher.
Nuffield gym membership.
England Cricket team for their signed photo.
Odeon cinema for tickets.
Surreal hair and beauty voucher.

Wilkinsons, Mansfield for photo frames, thank you Sir Ranulph Fiennes (my hero) for the signed book, Bear Grylls for your signed Scout photo (someone bought that off the winner for quite a sum), Lee Westwood for the signed photo and golf hat, and finally another hero of mine - James Cracknall - for your signed book; I'd have pinched it if I didn't already have two!

A special thanks to Advancis Medical, who not only donated lots of medical kit for our weary feet, but also gave us £500 - that really helped us with accommodation and fuel costs.

With regards to all the money raised, I could write a book on people who donated to our charities, or who bought raffle tickets ... but I can't, so here follows special thanks to people who really helped out:

To Ben, who helped raised money so we didn't have to pay for the entire event ourselves, the wives would have gone mad if we'd spent any more.

Thanks to all the guys at Thoresby Colliery who raised £700 ... brilliant effort.

Thanks to everyone at Doosan Power systems for raising £700; although I know a lot of it was due to my missus fluttering her eye lashes at you.

Thanks to Louise, Mark, Carol, Gary, Karen, Phil, Mum and Dad for taking a sponsorship form away with you and bringing me back lots of cash, even though you've done it all before for me.

Thanks to Ian, Ben and Aidy for selling zillions of raffle tickets and raising lots of money.

On behalf of Help for Heroes and The Amazon Breast Support Group (cancer awareness) ... I thank you all.

On a personal note, I thank my team mates - Ben, Aidy and Ian. I said at the start of this book that, selfishly, I used this race to provide not only a worthy event for you to take part in and raise charity money, but also something that would push my own limits in a way I have never done before, both physically and mentally. Not only did you rise to the challenge and complete some very gruelling races, you allowed me to achieve my personal ambitions and share these amazing experiences with you, to give us a bond of friendship to last a lifetime. And, naturally but not lastly, my running gear sponsor - Kurio Performance Ltd; www.kurioperformance.com.

My next thanks go to Saun Brown and Lee Huffer, my support crew. I said in my diary that I should have picked my SC better. Granted, I think it's better that you have people from a running background to help you, purely because they some idea of what you're going through, and respond to your needs better. The fact is, they did a cracking job. Each night we had place to sleep and something to eat. Through ups and downs we got there, and at the end of the event they weren't paid; could have left at any time, but decided instead to stay and put up with us weary, tired, snappy runners. They took a week out their own lives, using their own cash to get by. Regardless of ramblings in my diary, I truly thank you both. Grinners (private joke).

My final and most heartfelt thanks go to four special ladies, Suze, Jac, George and Hayley. I'm glad I can write this now; when I tried to say it on the day I started to well up. Between January and September 2011 our lives centred around running, and the Coast to Coast. Every day focussed the event, be it running for hours, racing, meetings about or planning for it. We couldn't have done it without the wives and girlfriends - supporting and not nagging us for disappearing for hours each day, or boring them to death talking about it. On a personal note, Hayley supported me all the way, even though it meant me being away for a week at the end. I don't know how they put up with us, especially Suze with a baby to look after, and, amazingly, George with a 1-week old when we departed.

Although they put up with all that, I hope it continues as I'm sure they've had enough by now - we continually bore them with tales of the event. Aidy is particularly bad, hauling out the map book and pointing to different locations - "George, look, we ran through there ..."
" Yes Aidy, I know."

Appendix A

Basic Training plan.

To begin with, I divided up the time line between start and finish. I drew a line with January at the start and September at the end - 9 months - and then decided that by month six I wanted the team to be comfortable with marathon distance, and when I say comfortable, I probably just mean 'used' to it. This in effect broke the training plan into two. I then had to decide what to do each side of the training programme.

January to June.
I had to get the team and I from 'Okay' runners (previous half marathon experience), up to a good marathon standard in six months, so I scheduled in three marathons in this time and planned mileage around them.

- Belvoir Marathon: March
- White Peak Marathon: May
- Cheviot fell race: June

This meant a stiff training schedule to ready the lads for a marathon by March; and taking into account a week off running before the race we had 9 weeks. Again, the simple approach was to break it up, consider - where you need to be before the race, where you are now, then simply fill in the gaps. This gives you your weekly long run target.

January			February			March		
8	10	12	14	15	16	16	18	19	26

Above is a simple line I drew up in my training diary. I put in the 8 mile point where we were, then marked the 19 mile mark where I wanted to be a week before our Belvoir marathon. From there I filled in the gaps as evenly as I could, and used this as a structure for a

65

training plan. Easy ... well, it's easy to write it up anyway. Now that we had a basic plan of what distance/s we needed to achieve each week, we squeezed in two other sessions per week - one speed and one medium / long distance run. Whilst on the subject I'll digress.

Speed sessions.
These are very important to maintain in your training programmes, especially if you're aiming for a marathon. Granted, if you move on to serious multi-day long distance runs, your training schedule will not allow you to keep up these sessions (see later), but whilst training for the single long distance event it's essential to maintain those speed sessions. They keep your legs strong and your CV system running smoothly and economically. Long distance running doesn't raise your heart rate and therefore doesn't really give it a work out ... but, you smash those hills out and boy ... your heart gets a workout.

March to June.
Once the first marathon was out the way I built up the training between March and June, keeping to the long weekly run (up to 18-19 miles) plus a speed session and a medium distance run (between 10 and 15 miles). Quite often, to keep the lads company, I'd run a long one with Aidy one day and repeat it the next day with Ben. I didn't mind; I felt I was getting my back-to-back training in early - but all it brought was injury ... the very reason I hadn't included it in the training plan originally. Runners ... we're all bloody idiots at some stage, we never listen to ourselves.

June to September.
Once the Cheviot Race was out the way in June I presented the new training plan. It looked bloody awful. Instead of 'total long distance runs' per week I listed 'time in hours' as the marker, and also how

many times per week. Although we'd be running for 7-12 hours a day for six days, I had no intention of training anywhere near that - it would simply result in injury, so settled for a 4 day running week. This would be plenty alongside a full time job.

July.

- 04-10: 2 / 2 / 2 / 2
- 11-17: 2.5 / 2.5 / 2 / 2
- 18-24: 2.5 / 2.5 / 2.5 / 2.5
- 25-31: 3 / 2.5 / 2.5 / 2.5

August.

- 01-07: 3 / 3 / 2.5 / 2.5
- 08-14: RACE WEEKEND (12-13th Grimsthorpe 70)
- 15-21: 3 / 3 / 3 / 3
- 22-28: 3.5 / 3 / 3 / 3
- 29-04: 4 / 3 / 3 / 3

September.

- 05-11: WIND DOWN & CHILL
- 12-18: RACE WEEK

As you can see, this is a 'grueller' of a training programme, and was followed almost religiously ... although maybe I did get ahead of myself with 4 x 3 hour runs after the Grimsthorpe 70.

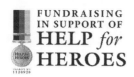

FUNDRAISING IN SUPPORT OF HELP *for* **HEROES**

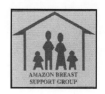

AMAZON BREAST SUPPORT GROUP

6 ULTRA MARATHONS
6 DAYS

COAST TO COAST

IN 6 DAYS

CONTENTS.

CHARITY AND RACE INFORMATION (PAGE 76 & 77)

DETAILED DAILY ROUTE DESCRIPTION

DIRECTIONS TO ROBIN HOODS BAY, PARKING (PAGE 84 & 85)

FINISH AREA, MAPS, (PAGE 86 & 87)

SUGGESTED FINISH TIME, CONTACT DETAILS (PAGE 87)

RESTAURANT DETAILS: TIMINGS, LOCATION (PAGE 88)

FUNDRAISING
IN SUPPORT OF
HELP *for*
HEROES

On consecutive days, we aim to run six ultra marathons in six days across the width of England along the Coast to Coast route. This will constitute running over 32 miles a day for the six days along a route which is usually done in two to three weeks. This equates to over 192 miles in less than a week! Whilst this is a huge challenge in itself, our bigger aim is to raise funds for two very worthwhile charities:

Help for Heroes was founded in October 2007 by Bryn and Emma Parry out of a desire to help wounded service men and women returning from Iraq and Afghanistan. In less than four years the charity has become nationally known and respected for its wonderful work with veterans. With many eminent individuals among its patrons, its message is simple:

"We are strictly non-political and non-critical; we simply want to help. We believe that anyone who volunteers to serve in time of war, knowing that they may risk all is a hero. These are ordinary people doing extraordinary things and some of them are living with the consequences of their service for life. We may not be able to prevent our soldiers from being wounded, but we can help them get better."

As Police Officers, we're occasionally required to put ourselves in harm's way in the line of duty, but this pales in comparison with the situations which young men and women from our armed services find themselves in on a daily basis. We believe their courage deserves our support.

Our other nominated charity is The Amazon Breast Support Group, and is significantly closer to home for us. Based in King's Mill Hospital in Nottinghamshire, it was founded by twelve breast cancer patients who felt that help for patients, beyond routine hospital medical care, was needed. From newly diagnosed patients to those discharged from hospital the charity offers help, advice and support. Few of us can be untouched by the trauma associated with a breast cancer diagnosis. This local charity provides invaluable support to women, and men, who are themselves living through the trials of the disease.

Day 1 (Mon 12th)

ST BEES TO ROSTHWAITE

START: St Bees (Beach)
Check point references

CP 1: Cleator (9 miles)   014 134

CP 2: Ennerdale Bridge, Moorend (6 miles)   077 158

CP 3: Slate Mine Visitors Centre (12 miles)   225 135

END: Rosthwaite (4.5 miles)   259 149

CAMPING BARN:
Dinah Hoggus, Stonecroft   259 150
Borrowdale, CA12 5XB
01768 774 301

POINTS TO NOTE:
Camping barn booked and paid for.

Total: 31.5 miles

Day 2 (Tues 13th)

ROSTHWAITE TO SHAP (32 miles)
Check point references

START: Rosthwaite   259 150

CP 1: Mill Bridge (A591) (8 miles)   335 091

CP 2: Patterdale ('P' on A592) (8 miles)   395 159

CP 3: Burnbanks (Naddle Bridge) (12 miles)   510 159

END: Shap (A6)   562 155

CAMPING:
Scott Newburn, Newing farm,   562 156
Main Street, CA10 3LX
01931 716 719

POINTS TO NOTE:
Campsite booked and paid for, including use of
showers.

Total: 32 miles

Day 3 (Wed 14th)

SHAP TO KELD (33.5 miles)
Check point references

START: Shap (A6)   562 155

CP 1: Orton (B6261) (9 miles)   624 080

CP 2: Ravenstonedale (Road) (6 miles)   694 065

CP 3: Kirkby Stephen (A685) (6 miles)   775 087

END: Keld (camp site) (12.5 miles) 887 014

CAMPING:
Heather & Steve Swann,
Park House Camp site   887 014
Bridge End, Keld, DL11 6DZ,
01748 886 549

POINTS TO NOTE.
Campsite booked but not paid for (inc.
electric hook up, £35 to be paid on day)

Total: 33.5 miles

Day 4 (Thu 15th)

KELD TO STREETLAM (34 miles)
Check point references

START: Keld   887 014

CP 1: Reeth (11 miles)   038 993

CP 2: Richmond (10.5 miles)   167 011

CP 3: Bolton-On-Swale (7.5 miles)   252 992

END: Streetlam (5.5 miles)   310 988

CAMPING: 337 987
The White Swan Inn,
Danby Wiske, Northallerton,
N Yorks, DL7 0NQ
Tel: 01609 775 131, mobile: 07742 735 343.

POINTS TO NOTE.
The Streetlam finish can be extended by approx 2
miles to Danby Wiske, where the campsite is based;
this will be dependent on the day, but either way the
support vehicle will be at Streetlam first.
Campsite booked but not paid for (inc electric hook
up), £33 to be paid on day.

Total: 34 miles (possibly 36 miles)

Day 5 (Fri 16th)

STREETLAM TO LION INN (32 miles) Check point references

START: Streetlam   310 988

CP 1: Road nr Renny Farm (9.5 miles)   416 010

CP 2: TK (Hollin Hill, Swainby), (7 miles)   493 008

CP 3: Road Parking (B1257), (7 miles)   573 035

END: Lion Inn (6.5 miles)   679 997

CAMPING:
The Lion Inn, Blakey Ridge,   679 997
Kirkbymoorside, N Yorks
YO62 7LQ
Tel: 01751 417 370

POINTS TO NOTE.

Booked but not paid for, £15 on day, no electric hook up, showers in pub.

Total: 32 miles (30 if start at Danby Wiske)

Day 6 (Sat 17th)

LION INN TO ROBIN HOODS BAY (29 miles)

START: Lion Inn   679 997

CP 1: Glaisdale (9 miles)   774 058

CP 2: A169 Sleights Moor P (7 miles)   885 043

CP 3: Hawsker (8 miles)   928 075

CP 4: Robin Hoods Bay North (5 miles) 951 055

END: ROBIN HOODS BAY FINISH 953 048
B&B. All parties with different setup.

POINTS TO NOTE.

CP4 is for changing into finishing kit. The end can
be subject to change depending on time, fatigue etc.
To shorten we will (after CP2 when we hit the B1416
GR 901 041), take the road route in, left and north on
A171, then R to Robin Hoods Bay at GR 923 046.

Total: 29 miles

DIRECTIONS TO ROBIN HOODS BAY

The majority of spectators will be travelling from the south. The best route is:

1.   A1(M) northbound

2.   At exit 44, take A64 towards York

3.   Keep on A64 around York towards Malton, Scarborough

4.   At Malton, take A169 towards Pickering, Whitby

5.   At Whitby take A171 towards Whitby, Robin Hoods Bay (carry on past Whitby)

6.   At Hawsker take left on B1447 Robin Hoods Bay.

Postcode for Robin Hoods Bay for your Satnavs: YO22 4RA.

Typical distance from Mansfield is: 124 miles.

Typical journey time from Mansfield is: 2 hours 12 minutes.

PARKING AT ROBIN HOODS BAY

As you come into Robin Hoods Bay off the B1447, you will hit a roundabout which puts you on Station Road leading to New Road. New Road leads you all the way to the finish line area.

There is official parking just prior to the roundabout, and also on New Road which is closer to the finish.

All websites advise that parking is not easy in Robin Hoods Bay, so please arrive early and have a drive round if you want to get as close to the finish as possible.

A lot of these car parks at Peak time / season will charge a minimum of £3 for 4 hours.

The finish ...

The route officially finishes at Robin Hoods bay outside a pub called 'The Bay Hotel'. This is right next to the sea and has an official plaque (inset) on it stating The Finish Line.

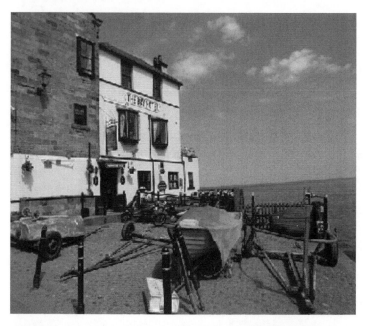

THE BAY HOTEL'S OFFICIAL ADDRESS IS:

The Dock,
Robin Hoods Bay,
WHITBY,
North Yorkshire
YO22 4SJ

Tel: 01947 880278.

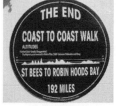

The Dock is located at the end of New Road with the junction of Kings Street. Attached is a map showing the Bay Hotel in relation to the route in from New Road with the junction of King Street.

SUGGESTED FINISH TIME

Each day our routine will be up at 6.00am and running for 8.00am. The final day is subject to change as the distance is 29 miles, which can be shortened if required. Also, if not all spectators are present, we'll wait just outside the bay before our final run in.

Saun Brown, our support driver will be keeping everyone updated as to our ETA.

I suggest an ETA of around 3.00pm - 4.00pm.

THE EVENING MEAL ... is booked for
7.00pm at **TRENCHERS RESTAURANT** in Whitby.

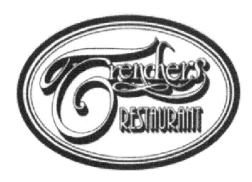

TRENCHERS
New Quay Road,
Whitby,
North Yorkshire,
YO21 1DH
email: enquiries@trenchersrestaurant.co.uk
Telephone: 01947 603212

A little about Trenchers:
Whitby Fish and Chips at Trenchers:

TRENCHERS Seafood Fish and Chips
Restaurant in Whitby is well known throughout the
North of England, especially in Yorkshire, for its fresh
traditional fish and chips menu served throughout the
day for lunch, high tea or evening dinner.

TRENCHERS Seafood Fish and Chips
Restaurant is situated in the centre of Whitby,
opposite the Whitby tourist office and Whitby railway
station, it is famous for its high quality fresh fish,
legendary light batters, bread-crumbed-and-floured
fish served by smart, courteous staff, guaranteeing
you a meal to remember.

DIRECTIONS
Simple directions would be travel to the Tourist office
or the railway station ... can't miss it.

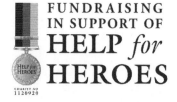

THANK YOU

Thank you, from all the team, for taking the time to come see us over the line. I'm positive the team will all be there at the finish in one way or another, maybe a little lighter, maybe a little tired or worse for wear, maybe missing a soul or two having left it somewhere in Cumbria, but we will be there.
Thanks again.

James.

A word from my running gear sponsor, Kurio Performance Limited:

Kurio Performance is pleased to support James Oliver on this, and all his expeditions.

Kurio custom made compression wear promotes faster, more efficient blood flow, ultimately helping James recover quicker, train harder, feel better, and potentially gain extra sessions in the gym.

Customized compression is not intended for the amateur athlete; rather for the serious competitor seeking the advantage. So, whilst everyone else is recovering in bed, come race day you will be out there making the difference.

Kurio - Designed and manufactured in the UK.
The ultimate in compression wear.
www.kurioperformance.com

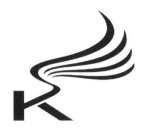

Printed in Great Britain
by Amazon